It Is NOT Luck

By AJ Berry

Books by AJ Berry
Non-Fiction
Times Past

The Terror Series
Non-Fiction
A Time of Terror
So It Was Written
Brothers in Arms

Out of Time Series
Fiction
Out of Time
In Her Time
Time for Healing
The Time Traveler's Children
The Time Traveler's Husband
Into The Time Slip
Stuck In Time
Twist In Time
Time for Love
Papa's Time
Time to Tell Mama
As Time Passes
Never Enough Time
Layers of Time
Time and More Time

Counting Series
Fiction
One for The Money
Two for The Show
Three to Make Ready
Four to Go
Five for The Fire

Revolutionary War Pension Series
Non-Fiction
By AJ Berry & James F. Morrison
Don't Shoot, Part 1
Don't Shoot, Part 2
Don't Shoot, Part 3
Don't Shoot, Part 4

It's A Distinct Choice.

"This poor old body!"

The lady was struggling for sure, she was trying to get down the steps at the church to go for the after church coffee and sweet treat. It was not easy for her to negotiate the steps; she was going very slowly and grumbling as she went.

"Sorry to hold you up! Just wait until you get this old!"

This litany went on and on. She made it down another step and I was getting impatient because every step brought a complaint and appeal for sympathy. It didn't seem she needed the entire broad staircase to get down the stairs and I wanted to go home.

"This poor old body! It's not good to get old. You have to be patient with me."

"Terrible to get this old, you'll see!"

Finally I exploded and said, "Just how old are you, how long do I have before I reach your stage?"

The lady told me, and she was about 10 years younger than I.

"How about you stop for a moment and let me past? You are nothing but a kid yet."

"Poor me, you are so lucky!"

"Luck has nothing to do with it."

I know it was not a nice thing for me to say, but I also knew that in her case, old age had very little to do with her problem. She was obese, not old, just very, very fat. Supposedly she was thin while she was courting her second husband and as soon as they married, she began to happily eat.

As I drove home, I thought about 10 years back in my own life. I was heavier 10 years ago than I used to be when I was younger, this I knew; I was still grieving for my husband and didn't really care about my appearance at all.

I knew it was time to make some changes, but I could put it off another day, but I knew it was going to happen. And it did for me, at last.

I think I had been marking time, just waiting to die; my father died at 62 and my husband at 65. Those numbers kept flashing behind my eye lids. Well, I passed those numbers and took out an option for 20 more years, not to just exist but to really live.

This part of life is really annoying!

It seems every time I go to the doctor's office I am faced with fat people. Usually there is a very obese one leaning over the intake window, too fat to stand up without leaning on the counter, and small as I am, I can't get past. All of them wear stylish sweat suits; (that's sarcastic) I guess sweat suits are all that fits them. They are loud in the waiting room, those fat people; complain about their lot in life, how difficult life is, and how much pain and suffering they have to go through. They claim that they can't help themselves and that they hardly eat anything. I can see the fat rolling of the top of the blue jeans and the men's' bellies hanging over the tops of their jeans as well. When I was younger, we wore clothing to cover it up more.

Whatever happened here? I see fat people wearing sweat suits that don't leave a bit to my imagination.

When I leave the doctor's office, why do I have another blocking the exit door to the doctor's office? The last time I had to wait until a woman moved and even then, I was careful I didn't get stepped on. Believe me it hurts to have a 300 plus something step on me. They claim I am too small for them to see. Really!

Why is it someone else's fault they are fat and in pain? I can't wait to get myself out of there. I move from chair to chair trying to escape the whining voices in the waiting room, I get a flash of fear that it might be contagious and then I begin to feel guilty for how well I feel. Are we a nation of people who won't take responsibility for our actions; do we lay awake at night trying to figure out who's fault it is that we have a problem?

I have noticed some people come out of the doctor's office in a really angry frame of mind, "The doctor told me to lose weight, now how dare he say that to me!" Actually an ex-friend told me this and I said, "Could be you need to lose weight?"

That made two people that person didn't speak to after the office call to the doctor.

Fat people like to sit near me on an airplane, or in crowded situations, they figure they are entitled to my space and worse yet; I usually get another fat person on the other side of me, which leaves me with less than half a seat. Those people think it is funny. Sometimes they ask me to please move for one reason or another, so they can have my seat if I am lucky enough to have a window seat or aisle seat.

There is a huge problem in the grocery store as well. My mother and I used to grocery shop together and both of us would leave the store grumbling about the big people who think we are not significant enough to walk around; they would head right for me and her with their carts and we had to jump out of the way. You might say that I should let them knock me down, but that can cause a world of hurt for me and injuries which might be permanent, some of those people already think they live in the world of entitlements, that they are better than the next person. I doubt my medical bills would be paid; they don't look wealthy to me.

Some people have knocked me down more than once and never stopped to apologize. Now when I see a person head for me, I put my hand in my pocket, thus making my elbow stick out, and then pick up my speed. This clips them in the ribs nicely, and they don't like it. I am satisfied to tell you that the ones who did this to me more than once, and received my treatment back; well, they haven't spoken to me since then or knocked me down.

I guess I am not always nice, but I have a problem, things just pop right on out of my mouth before I can stop them and then it lies there stinking. I guess it is the case on this particular subject.

Or could it be that the newly converted are the most self-righteous about it? I was overweight once myself. It was not just my appearance; I was having trouble moving about. When I got out of my recliner, I had to rock the chair back and forth enough to propel me forward in order to accomplish this task. I couldn't bend over well, my stomach met me part way down and I got out of breath over the smallest task.

My hips were giving me a lot of pain and it had been suggested to me by my doctor that I needed hip surgery; I also was having injections in my knees, they were giving me a lot of pain. I was about 60 years old, and feeling very old indeed.

And so I huffed and puffed about, trying to continue on with my life. All those around me sympathized, and reminded me I was getting old and entitled to having difficulty. What other pleasures are left in life at that age?

I say this is a choice, not luck; bad or good, at all. The path I chose was a difficult one; it is not easy to lose 50 pounds. All I can say is that you have to want to be thin more than eat a sweet for a fleeting second of pleasure. Look at that treat you are about to eat, you will want another shortly, guaranteed, and the pleasure will be fleeting with permanent guilt.

At the end of the day, can you say that you controlled yourself? If so, you can think with satisfaction about your excellent day.

There is no way around it, consume more than you burn, you wear it.

Every extra mouthful of food more than I needed would bring less for me to eat on the next day. I had to think about what I ate, was I hungry? Would what I want my food to do, help me or hurt me?

It was a long and difficult road. The plus part of it is that I rejoice when I garden now, I can easily bend over from my waist and do my gardening. It feels SO good! It has been about 10 years since I lost weight. I have energy, and the zest for doing things.

My joints don't have the severe pain they once had. This is huge for me, I couldn't believe the relief I got from the weight loss. Every pound impacts the joints and increases the arthritis pain; one pound brings 3-5 times more pressure on a joint, so 10 pounds of extra weight will bring 30-50 pounds of extra weight on the joints. That's a lot and very painful. Pick up 50 pounds and carry it around for an hour, it will hurt. Give your body a break.

In fact it's not just pain, the extra weight brings more wear and tear on the joints and osteoarthritis is just one of the problems overweight people develop.

I see so many in this village of ours who are overweight and struggling to get around, it makes me want to tell them the secret to feeling well again and full of life. We used to be told that it was normal to gain a few pounds for every year of life, but that no longer is a valid thought.

What types of foods are you eating?

The weight on the joints is not the only problem from food, the kinds of food you ingest are very important. Red meat is something I try to avoid as much as possible, I eat very few meals with red meat in it. I don't miss what I shouldn't have, I enjoy what I can eat, and there is a lot of that food available. It's a bit hard to find because all the STUFF is screaming at me every place I go.

I was amazed at a man checking out at Price Chopper, it was early morning and his man had several heaping carts of food. I checked out my groceries, and then peeked at his total; it was close to $500. Then I noticed what food he was buying, it was all prepared junk food. That made me feel heartsick for him and the family he was no doubt shopping for; he was overweight and no doubt the family was as well.

Sure you miss your old foods, but after a time you won't miss those foods. I find if I crave something, I want it often. But then when my circumstances changed, I didn't have the opportunity to eat those things and before long I didn't want that food again.

I know everyone thinks they have rights to do as they please, that I understand, but why do I have to pay for another persons weaknesses? Where is personal responsibility in this world?

This is the generation that might have our children die before we do; they are the first generation raised on junk food. The mother was working, and it was easier to buy junk food and the kids were happy with it. Turn on the TV too, keeps them quiet. This is a bad one way street; one brings on more of the other. The kids see the ads on TV; they sit and sit and eat and eat. Not good, and the habits continue throughout life.

I can't give you specific advice, but I can tell you about the process I went through to get myself healthy and lighter.

I do have a high and low number that I watch on my scale. Too thin is not good either, I have a 5 pound variance and make myself stay between 93-98 pounds. I am below 4' 9" unhappily, that seems to be my lot because I can't seem to grow. At the high end of the weight allowance, I know it's time for a correction, and I make myself do it at once. According to the height weight charts, I am still too heavy, but my body doesn't like to be lighter. A few times I dipped to 87 pounds, and that figure makes me nervous. The trick is to put some pounds on, but then to stop at the appropriate time.

Even at those weights, my joints complain at 98 pounds and coming down just a few pounds brings glorious relief.

Weigh yourself often; keep your goal in mind and an eye on your eating habits.

When I step on the scale at night and notice a weight gain, I reflect on what I ate or didn't eat. A four pound change in a day can be from several things for me. I drank a lot of water, or ate a lot of watery things, or I ate too much cheese and the salt in the cheese retained fluid for me. I weigh myself mornings to remind myself what I need to eat for the day. This seems important to me, I need to keep my eyes focused on my parameters. I have read that people who weigh themselves everyday lost more weight. As for myself, I can go badly astray in one short day. I weigh myself morning and evening, I need this crutch; and this habit goes back to high school.

When you eat is important!

I found that I can eat lightly in the mornings, and then eat a hearty lunch, after that only a very light snack, period. With this schedule, I don't seem to feel deprived. I know I process food more slowly than most people and with my small stature, I don't require the caloric intake others do. I know--I'm too short for what I want to eat.

Activity is important!

We as humans have made many changes to our lives in the past 200 years. I used to wonder how women could cook, churn butter, pop out a kid every other year, spin, weave, sew, tend to a garden and help with the heavy work, and so forth. How did they find the time to cook any meals?

I used to watch my grandmother catch a chicken, chop off its head, plunge it in boiling water, pull off the feathers, de-gut the chicken, remove the pin feathers, clean it well, cut it up and then fry the chicken. The rest of the meal was no easy task either. It was time consuming and took most of the day to get it all together.

Then I realized that they didn't cook back then, they only did it for special occasions. Those folks only ate to stay alive and not live to eat as we do. An old nursery rhyme popped into my head one day and pulled me up short!

Peas porridge hot, peas porridge cold,
Peas porridge in the pot, nine days old.

AHA! They didn't cook either! Whatever they had to eat was thrown in the pot to stew over the hearth fire. Sometimes they had meat and sometimes not. Now that is a huge change for humans and a startling realization for me. They ate to stay alive, and ate only what was available to eat, which was not much. The body stored fat for those lean times; it is what it is programmed to do. The rich folks could eat everything in sight, but not the poor folks. I think we are programmed to want to eat and store up some fat for the time of little.

With insatiable appetites, and plenty of easy to purchase prepared food, we are a disaster.

Once I was a yo-yo dieter and struggled to lose weight and keep it off. I found all kinds of ways to excuse myself.

Burn an extra 1,000 calories a day!

My oldest son read this booklet and reminded me to mention exercise. He runs 5-7 miles a day and this exercise is perfect for him since he doesn't know where in the world he might be or what time of day. If it is the middle of the night, he runs in a secure area, otherwise he maps out his runs along the streets near his home. To be sure he runs enough; he uses an Excel spread sheet on his computer to keep the tally.

His epiphany occurred one day when he stepped on the scale and realized he weighed 200 pounds with a double chin. He told me he was emotionally unprepared to weigh over 200 pounds and started running. With his plan he can eat everything he likes to eat. He has tried to convert me, but my joints can't take the pounding.

Let's see if I can remember my excuses.

A meal was what I ate before I could have dessert. When I planned a meal, I planned dessert first.

When I get to a certain weight, then I can eat. And I did so; what I put on in a flash came off at a snail's pace. I figured probably because I had to make up for my past sins and I wasn't noticing all I put in my mouth.

I'm buying the candy for the kids. (Don't do that, don't bring it home, then you won't eat it.) I tried to hide the goodies but I knew where the bodies were buried and that was not a good plan. I couldn't rest until I ate the whole thing.

Go ahead, eat it, you deserve it.

I need to keep my strength up.

I ate it before I realized it.

Or I forgot I ate that food.

Just one more won't matter. I'll be careful the rest of the day, won't eat a thing.

I'm already over the calories, what matters? Just eat it and hope it doesn't show.

I'll make up for it tomorrow.

Fats and carbohydrates.

Those two things for me at least, seem to trigger the eating frenzy, so I try to avoid them. It will take days to remove the damage they cause. Eat enough to be healthy but don't look for extra fatty things. For me Italian foods trigger this eating frenzy, so I plan what I want to order before I got into the restaurant. Then I am aware of the ensuing problem and can head it off.

Handy convenience stores.

Being on the road is a tough one too. So much of what we eat is snack food when we are gone all day with no time for a regular meal. Then too, I would think about food while driving. I had time to stop at Stewart's or Cumberland Farms for a treat. Be careful, what I see there are small amounts of food, high calorie, and so much is not healthy food. Mostly those foods trigger my eating frenzy.

I avoid chocolate, gives me heartburn. Avoid nuts, they tend to get trapped in those nasty pockets in my intestines and gives me belly pain. I try to stay away from sugary things. I can taste the artificial flavoring in too many things and they blot out the taste of the food. Some things are made almost totally out of artificial things, even some plastics are used.

Eating on the run.

There is not much left to eat while on the bus run break, so I usually get a small dip of ice cream and that seems to help and not trigger the eating reflex. A good lunch or snack that fills me up is a 6 inch sub from Subway. I really feel full and satisfied with that amount of food. Eat slowly, it takes time for your brain to register you are full, so you should eyeball your food and estimate how much will satisfy you and then stick to it. The other way is a few miserable hours to feel too full.

Artificial flavoring.

For me now, eating a large meal of artificially flavored foods can make me sick. My body won't accept it and that is a help to better eating habits. If I just have to have a treat, I buy it and then usually eat just a little of it. The first bit is delicious and after that it goes rapidly downhill. The coating in my mouth and the lingering distaste of the snack render it disgusting to me.

All calories are not alike.

As an example, a week or so ago, I made strawberry short cake. I knew the calories in what I was eating, so figured I could indulge and eat my fill. I was appalled to see I gained 3 pounds during the course of that day. I ate in volume what I normally eat, and in caloric count, but my body didn't appreciate my great "Sacrifice", and showed me. Games don't pay off in that department. I need "good" calories.

Keep track of the calories.

Be aware of the good calories and the not so good calories. A candy bar should never replace your lunch in spite of your caloric intake. I know better, but sometimes I just gotta eat those things. I always regret it; the treat did not give me much satisfaction by evening when I stepped on the scale along with the terrible heartburn. That meant I would have to be doubly careful of what I ate the next day.

Let's talk about those "0" calorie sodas. If they don't put on weight how come I lost 15 pounds when I stopped drinking diet soda? I drink water, lots of cold water. It was hard to part from the diet soda, but I don't retain fluid like I once did. Besides those things are horribly expensive. I am almost afraid to drink some diet soda for fear I will become obsessive about it again.

Sugar Free.

Or even low sugar foods. Check the labels, I find that the sugar substitutes will make me want a lot more and mentally when you read the label you figure you can eat two times as much food. Sometimes the low sugar difference is so miniscule, that you are better off eating the sugar variety.

MIA, Missing in action.

I no longer seem to be able to eat foods I once ate and digested with no problem. When I argued about it, my body made it very clear I could not eat that stuff any longer. I got sick from it, which was helpful. I read someplace that we have fewer digestive bacteria and enzymes in our digestive tract than when we are younger.

Phew!!!

Bloating and gas make me unfit for human society, so I avoid those foods as well. Now the regular ones such as cucumbers and baked beans don't bother me at all, most everything else gives me gas. We all have different bodies and have to treat them differently. I try to plan my poison carefully.

Not True.

Don't think losing weight is easier for a small person, it comes off a lot harder because there is less to begin with, I would guess. My body is very stubborn about the whole thing and it makes me unhappy. It seems once I hit the weight gain button, it doesn't want to stop it; that's why I set the parameters for maximum and minimum.

Calories in, calories used.

You have to eat less than you burn in other words. Exercise can assist you here, just remember eat more than you remember and then you burn a lot less than you think you do, so don't count on getting 16 hours of exercise a day, be reasonable in your assumptions. I know that in order to lose weight, since I don't burn as much as a larger person, I have to eat about 700-800 calories a day. I drink a lot of water with my meals and that helps me feel full.

A fast way to lose weight.

At one point in my life for various reasons, I was forced to eat the very same thing day after day. I no longer looked forward to eating; my taste buds were bored to death. Eating didn't become something I did for pleasure, but I ate because I had to have food to survive. I ate only what I needed and not a bite more. If you try this easy fix, make sure the foods you select are good for you and you have a balanced diet.

How much raw or uncooked food do you eat?

Cooking destroys too much of the valuable nutrients in the food. I have read that 51% of our daily consumption must be RAW, not cooked or else the body will react with white blood cells and treat cooked food as an invader. Worse yet, the deficit builds up over time. This is interesting. A close friend of mine had a high white blood count and the doctor couldn't figure out where she had the infection. I suggested she might think about this, eat more raw foods. I noticed that when I do this, my pain level is much lower and I have more energy. Cooking food, especially vegetables, destroys a lot of the protein in the food.

Misleading labels.

Have you ever picked up a pre-packaged food and read the low caloric count on the label? Whoa! I have fallen for this trap myself! Notice first how many servings and the size of those servings for those low calories. That candy bar which is 4 inches long might list several servings, thereby giving you a misleading caloric figure. If you eat it while you are hungry, before you know it you have put away a full day of calories and will still feel hungry.

Feeling full!

My life changed when I lost my job and so did my eating habits. Before I had so little time to eat, I ate things with more calories in them while on the run. My life changed and then I was a constant companion to my refrigerator and my clothes got tight.

Time to rethink this whole thing and then shift gears, this had to stop. If you eat a high calorie candy bar, you might have 400 calories and feel unsatisfied probably because the candy bar doesn't occupy much space in your stomach. I didn't connect this until my favorite food season rolled around, August and September. I call it "eat all you want season"; a lot of delicious raw foods are available during this time. I can put away a huge cantaloupe by myself, and then follow it with fresh tomatoes and so forth. I was stuffed and didn't care to eat anything more because my stomach was full and I didn't feel deprived. This made me do some more research. I found I could eat double to four times the amount of raw food to get the nutrients I needed. I began eating all I wanted, and found that I actually lost weight, though at first it looked like I had gained because of the weight of the food. For instance a large juicy cantaloupe weighs several pounds, etc., and this shows on the scale. Eventually it will level out. Remember to drink a lot of water, all day long!

Where's the diet you might ask?

Not here, you should consult your doctor about that one. I don't like those things for me, the amount is far more than I can begin to eat and eating that amount of food would put more weight on me. One size doesn't fit all or as they say now, one size fits most. Every person's body seems to come with its own set of rules, you need to listen you what your body has to say to you—even then you need to weigh that with common sense and what works for you.

My granddaughter scolded me once and said, "Gram you need to eat 2,000 calories a day, that's the minimum. I can't consume that much, I need to stick to 1,000 to 1,200 calories a day and to lose weight I have to go to about 800 a day. That's a tough situation!

What's in it for me?

Even a relatively small weight loss will help you a lot, but that makes it easier to slide back to old habits. Why not go for all the weight you should lose while you are in the mood, that way it will show the world the new you and bring even greater benefits. The easiest part is taking it off, keeping it off is harder. Alcoholics stop drinking, but we all have to eat. You need to learn to get used to a new type of eating, one that will make it easier for you to continue on with your new life. The end all isn't to consume the best tasting food, it is to become healthier. The surprise will be once you adjust, you will prefer the new type of food and eating. Don't allow for a tiny slip, it can trigger that old frenzy once more and you can gain a lot of weight in just TWO days.

When you go ON a diet, what happens when you go OFF a diet?

Having a goal and meeting it is a great thing, but when you are on a diet, sooner or later you have to live back in the real world. I do better on working around things that I like to eat but in moderation. For instance don't just eat one food, some use the fad diets and they can cause health problems from not eating a balance of foods you need. I'm thinking about the Broccoli Diet, the Grapefruit Diet, and so forth. Make plans for the time you leave the diet; will you return to the old eating patterns?

Ah, that TV and the sofa, and the bed.

They are all no, no's for food consumption. You need to somehow alter that pattern of unconscious eating. Do not eat before bedtime, which is the worst time I think to consume food, it doesn't go away overnight. Perhaps use some exercise while watching TV? Join an exercise group? Make a personal rule to only eat at the table with a full place setting of plate, tableware, napkin? That way you will realize how much and what you are eating. The bed is always a no, no. If you have acid reflux, this is not good either. I like at least 6-8 hours between spoon and sleep.

Find an absorbing hobby, then use that to stall eating something. Usually the urge will go away. It is an urge, not hunger that is motivating you. Old habits die hard.

Acid Reflux.

I didn't think I had acid reflux; after all I was eating long before I went to sleep at night so I wouldn't have acid come up in my throat, in my ears and out my nose. How that would hurt!

What happened was I improved it, but didn't solve it. I went to a doctor about fixing my broken nose and she looked at my throat and pronounced, "Acid Reflux". Of course Dr. Berry (me) argued with her. She went on to explain that it was the silent type and that I still had the problem. "40% of Americans have this problem, so it is not a wild guess that you have it. Your throat is cooked."

For most of my life, I was told I had asthma and took a lot of drugs for it. Every specialist said I most surely had asthma but I complained the asthma medicines didn't do much for me. I wheezed, I rattled, I coughed up lots of nasty stuff, my sinuses were blocked, my ears were blocked and I had bad balance problems. I was a hunk of human misery for about 30-40 years. Specialists kept throwing more and more drugs at the problem which caused more problems. My blood pressure was high, I couldn't sleep, my heart pounded, etc.

Wow, what a revelation to be told I had acid reflux. She was right, when I eat something naughty and forget to take one of those famous drugs that control acid reflux; I have problems for a few days such as a lot of phlegm in my throat and the accompanying problems.

I threw away my nebulizer, my inhalers, and all the things I took to control my symptoms. In all I counted 6-8 drugs that I no longer use.

If you even suspect you have this problem, better have this situation checked out by your doctor, and then do as he or she suggests.

Try it; you will learn to like it.

I find junk food pretty disgusting now. I used to hate to eat vegetables, but once I started to eat them in a determined way and filled up with them, I began to feel better and after time I learned to like them. Spinach and vinegar for instance, that was the absolute pits to eat for me, and now it is a treat. It didn't happen overnight, but it happened. I never thought I would like getting up early for a job or for anything, but I did. It took quite a bit of time and eventually I got used to getting up early and finally I got sleepy earlier in the evening. I rather like this change, so I am keeping it even though I am not working outside my home, though I get up a little later than I had to for work. The same change applies to eating habits, keep at it and it will change.

Mostly my food eating habits consist of vegetables, fish, breads, salads, etc. Very little red meat and a lot of fish or salmon with chicken. Sometimes I just have a huge tossed salad with the works for a meal.

Your tastes can change.

This is not an overnight thing, and I try not to remind myself how I used to enjoy eating some foods. I naturally go for the right foods now, but still have to control my portions. I used to have a mouth full of sweet teeth as the saying goes, but now I turn my nose up at that stuff. Be ruthless, cut off eating those things totally, just a little is too much, so go cold turkey, it is easier. No sweets. You will begin to think about regular foods. Make sure you are not eating artificial foods. I bought a bunt cake mix a few months back, and fixed it to eat. To my horror, all I tasted was the artificial flavoring; what a turn off.

Salt is another thing you can do without.

This one took a few weeks, but then when I ate "regular" food, I noticed the salt and that I didn't like the taste of food with much salt. Another added bonus was that the excess fluid left my body.

Feeling deprived?

The one food I crave is cheese; I think if I had to pick one food I could eat for life, it would be cheese. Now cheese is a bad food for me, but I learned to limit my intake. Once I start on a cheese kick, I can eat a one pound brick of cheese in two days and then I have the excess fat to burn and the salt with the accompanying weight retention. That is one reason I weigh myself every day, I need to know if I am retaining fluid and that normally means I was eating too much cheese.

I'm not the only cheese face in the house, my dog loves it too. He can be three rooms away, napping, and once he hears the cheese drawer in the refrigerator open, he is right next to me, wagging his tail in a hopeful fashion. I know the signs well.

Use a smaller plate!

This is a simple adjustment, use a smaller plate to eat from, your plate can still be full but somehow you don't feel you are eating less. No second helpings are allowed. It takes time for you to feel full, so simply wait about a half hour and you will feel satisfied whereas if you have a second portion you will be uncomfortable in a half hour. You can adjust, your stomach can adjust, and most of all, your mind can adjust.

I dislike a huge plate filled with food placed in front of me. In the restaurants, the meals are huge and I don't go back to any place where I can't get a child's portion of food. I don't care if they charge me the same as for an adult portion; I hate to waste food and dislike all that food staring at me.

If you have to eat food in social situation, use portion control and only fill your plate ONCE. If you are served food, such as in a restaurant, use the Jackie O. trick. Cut everything in half and just eat a half portion. Lately even the child's portion is too big, forget the senior portions, they are still enormous. In my favorite restaurant I found I could order a baby size and when that grew to be too large, I now order a PREEMIE portion.

Restaurants are serving larger and larger portions of food, and America is demanding it as well.

To add flavor to your food, add sauces, spicy and hot, that will wake up your taste buds and help you adjust to a healthier diet.

My idea is not to just live longer, but to live longer going full steam ahead.

My goal is to keep out of the doctor's office and feel well for most of my remaining years. How would you like the idea of feeling fit, being able to run, and keeping yourself out of the nursing home? Now that was an eye opener for me. I exercise at the nursing home in the cold months and can see what happens to those my age who are obese. There are notable exceptions, but mostly the rule applies here. Eat for sport and live there. Too many my age are immobile and ill, I want to stay out of there.

What a goal some people have, eat all you can, get as fat as you can, feel sorry for yourself, and end up helpless in the nursing home or die from a horrible disease brought on by poor eating habits.

Hang on and die for the holt as they said in the Revolutionary War. MAKE IT HAPPEN.

This is indeed war. You have to want the benefits more than you want to eat for temporary satisfaction.

You can see I spend a lot of time thinking about food as we all do. Perhaps there are those who say I use self-hypnosis, or am I just being realistic about it?

Other triggers that I don't understand because I never had to deal with them are smoking and alcohol usage and/or addiction. I can add coffee to that list too. When I was 20, and we were close to marriage, my mother-in-law-to-be sat me down and said I had to drink coffee.

"You'll love this", she said as she poured cream and sugar into the cup. "You won't even taste the coffee."

I drank one swallow and I shuddered and gagged and then threw it up. That was the end of that subject. I don't even like mocha flavored ice cream, candy, or cakes. That is the way it is for me. My body is helpful with many things, it has simply caused me to stop wanting or liking certain foods, such as chocolate. I suppose I could argue with it and start eating it slowly, but I like it the way it is now. Occasionally I want chocolate and then I will buy something with artificially flavored chocolate, that reinforces the dislike and I don't want it again for a long time. No sense treating my taster, I don't see that I need to get the best to encourage my bad habit.

Don't think about food, change the subject.

Get yourself absorbed in something you enjoy, postpone the food thoughts. You will be surprised how much of the day you can get through this way when you first begin your journey. Hold off for one hour, and keep extending it. This is how I handle hard things; I can do anything almost for an hour at a time.

Donuts and so forth.

We live in a world filled with delicious donuts. I turn my nose up over them and feel my stomach doing likewise. I used to love donuts, a lot of them.

One night as I was on my way home I stopped and bought a dozen glazed donuts or doughnuts as they once were called. I ate one after the other until the whole box was gone. That solved that problem, I never ate another donut, I over dosed on them is what happened. The biggest problem this left me with is that people take it personally when I refuse coffee and when I refuse donuts. I hurriedly walk away from both of those things. I won't let others shame me into eating something I don't like, and they do take that one personally, it must be un-American. Everyone loves donuts.

Cook for yourself.

I package meals in the right proportions for myself and freeze them. Then I cook for the others in the family who don't like my foods.

So many diseases are linked to obesity; if you are 40% overweight you will have double the chance to die prematurely as a normal weight person.

At the end of the day, do you remember what you ate? Unlikely, so in the overall scheme of things, what did you do for your body? Help it live or help it die? Your choice.

Do you want heart disease, stroke, high blood pressure, diabetes, cancer, gout, sleep apnea, breathing problems? Some of these things will improve, some will go away. The win on this one is huge.

Those famous dieter's meals.

Let's talk about the dieter's meals, the name of which shall remain nameless. You have seen them all and I have no doubt they taste as good as they look. Are you going to continue buying that plan for the rest of your life? They figured out how to make things low calorie, but will you bother cooking that way? They don't break your craving for certain foods, think about the course you wish to pursue very carefully.

This is really about changing your eating habits and eating foods with healthy ingredients. When I hear these advertisements, I hear a celebrity talk about eating this yummy dessert and that yummy treat, all of which are usually high calorie when homemade or purchased in the store. I am suspicious as to how exactly they make these packages, what are they putting in that is low cal? Is if a natural substance or man-made or even plastic? Are you going to choose that way of life and gain it all back, or are you going to learn a better way to good health?

Belly surgery.

Everyone wants to continue their pleasures but not pay for their eating sins. I say that cannot happen.

The easy answers it seems to me, come with huge risks and many who have the surgery have some terrible side effects. A friend of mine ended up with a bowel obstruction (surgery) and a detached retina from all the vomiting. He's blind in one eye and worse yet; he can't control his appetite and is gaining it all back. Your eating habits need to change; this is not a magic answer.

My weight loss?

At one point it was about 60 pounds and now I maintain it at the 50 pound level. I lost 1/3 of me and I feel so much better; I have a LOT less pain, more energy, and I can move so much easier. Watch me garden by just bending over; I can work hours that way now. Love it. This year is marking my 10th year of losing that weight and I plan to keep it off. It is more difficult for a shorter person to lose weight; our bodies don't burn as much as a taller person.

Make changes one at a time, and then go on to the next change. It will help you and your body adjust to the new lifestyle.

Ultimately it is your choice; you have to want to be healthy more than you want to eat your favorite treat. Your choice entirely. Don't even think "I'll diet until I drop the weight and then I can eat what I want again." This is a lifetime, lifestyle changing event. If I did it, you can too. It is NOT easy at all. Say farewell to those things you eat and don't look back.

Eat yourself well.